Gateway to Nutrition

Resources for Food Assistance Agencies

Table Of Contents:

Dedicated to the Gateway Gaston's partner agencies-
Thank you for making our community a better place.

Chapter 1: Introduction

If you are reading this, you are involved with the charitable food system in some way. Maybe you are the director of a food assistance agency (FAA), a board member, a volunteer, or simply interested in how charitable food is distributed to help your neighbors. Your agency may provide nonperishable items with a food pantry, serve prepared meals, and/or ensure healthy foods like fruits and vegetables are available to everyone. No matter what role you play, it is important work. If you picked up this book, you are someone who is out to change the world, or, at least, a small part of it that belongs to you. The first point of this book is to say thank you. The world needs more givers, changemakers, and people fighting for justice. The world needs more people like you.

As we all know, food is one of the basic needs for human life. Without enough food, life cannot continue. Therefore, when food is inaccessible or in short supply, people must put all their mental and physical energy into obtaining it. When you help people obtain food, you empower them to allot energy towards improving their lives.

It is not simply a can of beans, a meal, or a box of vegetables. It is a resource. A crucial resource with the power to change someone's world for the better.

These pages are intended to encourage and empower, because food assistance is essential to the health of a community. This book discusses issues that commonly affect FAAs, such as barriers, food distribution models, food safety, nutrition, and cost-effectiveness. It provides resources that help to combat these issues, including information about food insecurity and food deserts, a guide to food safety, recipes, nutrition education tools, tips for delicious meals on a limited budget, and ideas for improving the nutritional quality of the food you provide. In addition, it is a collection of interesting ideas to fuel your imaginations as you continue to develop your service to the community.

Every FAA is unique and thus, by nature, not everything in this book will apply to you. You will find some sections in this book useful, while others will reiterate information you already know. That's fine. The goal is to create a resource that everyone can find helpful and inspiring. Consider this a book of suggestions, not an action plan.

The world of charitable food systems is always evolving. We are constantly facing new problems and brainstorming solutions. Improving the charitable food system requires the collaboration of a community of people with unique knowledge, ideas, and experiences. Please reach out with any thoughts, questions, feedback, or ideas by email at laurel@laureledavis.com. I would love to have a conversation with you.

Always remember that you are doing amazing work and building a brighter future for our community. The world needs you. Please keep going.

Chapter 1.5: Defining Key Terms

A few key terms must be defined so that everything discussed later makes sense.

According to the UCONN Rudd Center for Food Policy and Obesity, the **charitable food system** is the collective network of organizations and agencies, such as food banks, food pantries, food kitchens, and others, that provide food at no cost. Other names include the emergency food system or food banking system (the Rudd Center). Throughout this book, charities, agencies, nonprofit organizations, and houses of worship that provide food to people in need are each referred to as a **food assistance agency** (**FAA**). The goal is to create an all-encompassing term that can accurately describe a wide array of agencies, from crisis relief organizations to small food pantries to homeless shelters. These agencies have one thing in common- they give food assistance.

Next, it is important to understand food banks and food pantries, and the differences between them. Food banks and food pantries are two different types of organizations that are each vital to the charitable food system. However, the terms are often used interchangeably, causing confusion. In essence, the difference between food banks and food pantries is *where they exist within the supply chain.*

According to the Feeding America Hunger Blog, a **food bank** functions like a warehouse, storing food donated by producers, retailers, and restaurants in mass quantities. In addition, they connect sources of food directly with partner FAAs (Waite). While food banks may lead small, secondary programs that DO directly distribute food to clients, their primary goal is to facilitate the delivery of a steady supply of food to their partner FAAs (Waite).

A **food pantry** distributes the groceries supplied by a food bank directly to the clients who consume them (Waite). Food pantries are the face of the operation, and the organization with which the clients come into direct contact.

Food kitchens are agencies that serve prepared meals. A more common term is "soup kitchen," but not all of these agencies exclusively serve soup. They may distribute a variety of dishes, such as hot meals, sandwiches, or breakfast foods. Food kitchen, once again, is more all-encompassing.

Lastly "**clients**" refer to those who utilize food assistance. Other words you may see or use in place of this could be "neighbors" or "community members." These are the people who benefit from accessing an FAA's services. "Clients" is used in this book because it is a common term in the charitable food system. However, challenge yourself to consider which term is most dignifying for the people you serve. Words can be used as a tool to build people up. Language is powerful; use that power to empower

Chapter 2: The Problem

Food assistance agencies (FAAs) work to make healthy food available for everyone, addressing several issues in the community in which they are located. Two key issues are **food insecurity** and **food deserts**. Both are interrelated; both have long lasting negative effects on health and well-being.

The USDA Economic Research Service (ERS), defines food security as "access by all people at all times to enough food for an active, healthy life" ("Food Security in the U.S."). Levels of food security lie across a spectrum of four ranges: **high food security, marginal food security, low food security,** and **very low food security** ("Definitions of Food Insecurity"). High and marginal are considered **"food secure"** while low and very low are considered **"food insecure"** ("Definitions of Food Insecurity").

Households with high food security have zero barriers to food. Marginal food secure households have minor indicators of concern, such as fear of food running out, but little to no indication of reduced food quality or quantity. Households with low food security may reduce *quality, variety, or desirability*, but do not need to reduce the *quantity* of food they eat. Thus, low food security was once called "food insecurity without hunger." The lowest level of food insecurity is very low food security. In these households, one or more members have disrupted eating patterns and reduced food intake due to a complete lack of resources. In the past, it was referred to as "food insecurity with hunger" ("Definitions of Food Insecurity"). Both low and very low food insecurity can have a severe impact on the physical, mental, and emotional health of adults and children alike.

Low access areas or **food deserts**[1] are geographical areas where access to healthy and affordable food is limited ("About the Atlas"). There are several means by which food deserts are measured. The ERS defines these in one-half and one-mile demarcations for urban areas, and ten and twenty-mile demarcations for rural areas ("About the Atlas"). Census data is combined with results from the American Community Survey and a list of supermarkets to produce the Food Access Research Atlas, a free tool that shows geographical food access indicators across the United States ("About the Atlas"). It is housed on the ERS website. The link can be found in Chapter 2 resources.

---

[1] The ERS once called these "food deserts" but now uses "low access." This book uses "food deserts" because this term is more familiar to the general population.

Food insecurity and food deserts are detrimental to a person's health because they can result in poor nutrition. Both food insecurity and low food access can be caused by low income, as poverty is more prevalent in food desert tracts than non-food deserts (Dutko et. al. 11).

Most people consider food insecurity and food deserts on a national or global scale. However, these challenges can be observed right in the community of Gaston County. The problem is national and global, yet also local and personal. Here are a few important data points about Gaston County, NC from Feeding America's "Mind the Meal Gap" data and the Food Access Research Atlas:

- **14.3%** of Gaston County citizens were food insecure in 2019 (Gunderson et. al.).
- In total, **31,330** people were food insecure in Gaston County in 2019. Of these, **9,370** were children, placing the childhood food insecurity rate at **18.8%** (Gunderson et. al).
- **25** census tracts in Gaston county have a significant portion of residents living either 1/2 mile (for urban areas) or 10 miles (for rural areas) from the nearest supermarket ("Food Access Research Atlas").
- Of these tracts, **14** are at least 1 mile (urban) or 20 miles (rural) away from a supermarket ("Food Access Research Atlas").

Figure 1 and Figure 2 are images from the *Food Access Research Atlas*, depicting data from Gaston County:

Figure 1: Depicts census tracts in which a significant portion of residents live further than 1/2 mile (urban) or 10 miles (rural) from the nearest supermarket.

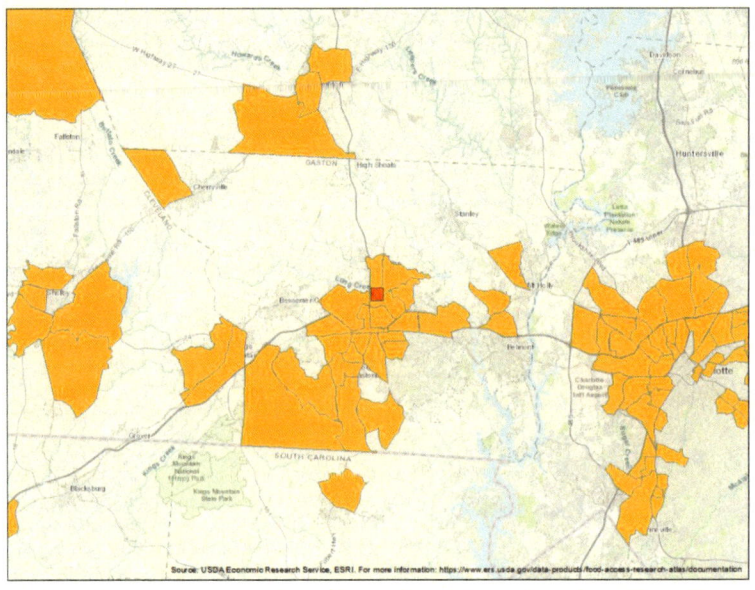

Figure 2: Depicts census tracts in which a significant portion of residents live further than 1 mile (urban) or 20 miles (rural) from the nearest supermarket.

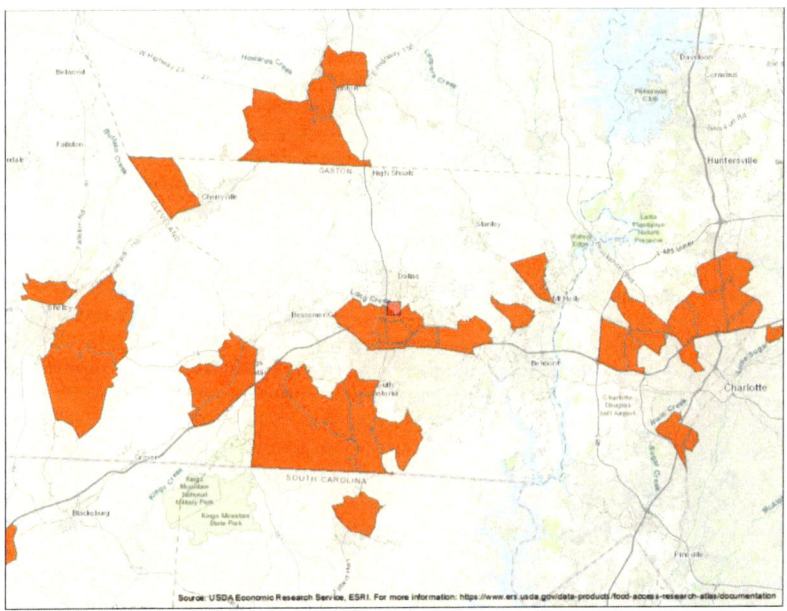

Images accessed from the USDA-ERS Food Access Research Atlas on 11/09/2021, with permission from Alana Rhone.
https://www.ers.usda.gov/data-products/food-access-research-atlas/go-to-the-atlas/.

FAAs are doing much needed work in Gaston County, helping neighbors struggling with food insecurity or living in food deserts. By increasing access to nutrition, FAAs help the community become stronger and healthier. The solution to food insecurity and food deserts begins with you.

Chapter 3: The Challenges

FAAs throughout the United States commonly face similar challenges. Many have effectively addressed some or all of these, others struggle to find solutions given their unique circumstances. Reexamining issues now may mitigate or even prevent issues from resurfacing in the future. This chapter summarizes several common challenges and serves as a preview of the ideas and resources throughout the rest of the book.

Organizational Assessment:

Chapter 4 contains an organizational self-assessment that FAAs might use to understand themselves better. The assessment is a tool that will help FAAs to pinpoint their own attributes, rules, and operation systems. In addition, FAAs may use this assessment to celebrate their successes, identify places where they would like to improve, and solidify goals for their future.

Barriers:

FAAs may struggle to meet the needs of the community, simply because their target demographic does not utilize their food assistance. There are almost as many possible barriers as there are potential clients. Barriers may be invisible or clearly evident. Ultimately, barriers prevent FAAs from helping people.

One example of a group facing barriers includes people described as "low food secure." These people must sacrifice dietary quality and desirability to have enough food ("Definitions of Food Insecurity"). Because these potential clients have *enough* food, they may not seek food assistance. They may even feel guilty, believing they are taking resources from neighbors who "need food more." However, additional dietary variety would improve health, stress levels, and quality of life for these potential clients. FAAs are truly excellent resources for these individuals.

Because many factors can be barriers, the solutions must be highly individualized for the FAAs and even for clients. Many FAAs have observed barriers and adapted accordingly in the past. Chapter 5 explores common barriers and introduces ideas to overcome them.

Food Distribution Models:

The way an FAA distributes food is part of its' "fingerprint" - a unique aspect that differentiates it from others in the community. Methods of distributing food are as diverse as FAAs themselves, but there are two general models, specifically in food pantries: the standardized box model and client-choice model. Chapter 6 discusses both, along with the benefits and drawbacks of each.

Mobile Food Pantry Model and Sample Stock:

The Gateway Gaston is working on an exciting new project- a mobile food pantry model. We are hopeful that this model will help effectively address food deserts in Gaston County. It involves distributing bagged "meal kits" made with easy recipes and healthy ingredients. Chapter 6 also contains a mobile food pantry sample stock based on these meal kits. The recipes for the meal kits are under Recipes in resources.

Food Safety:

No one intentionally allows foodborne illness to happen. Everyone has experienced foodborne illness, whether from the pasta salad at a potluck, unrefrigerated leftovers, or from a poorly sanitized restaurant. In many cases, foodborne illnesses cause brief sickness. Those affected might take a day off work then move on with their lives. However, for others, especially vulnerable populations such as children, the elderly, and those with compromised immune systems or chronic diseases, foodborne illness is especially dangerous.

Food safety is always of utmost importance, but particularly in food assistance agencies. Statistics show that many food-insecure individuals deal with high rates of chronic disease and limited access to medical care (see Chapter 7 for these statistics). Food safety must be an absolute priority within FAA operations, just as within their commercial counterparts including restaurants and grocery stores. Basic food safety standards and information can be found in Chapter 7.

Nutrition:

Eating healthy is essential. Proper nutrition prevents chronic disease, improves daily mood, increases energy levels, and much more. Nutrition deeply impacts health and overall quality of life. Unfortunately, barriers exist that prevent food-insecure individuals from eating healthfully. These barriers result in clear health consequences. Proper nutrition is a human right, so FAAs should take steps to improve nutrition for clients. Nutrition strengthens the health of clients and the community.

Chapter 8 summarizes basic nutrition information from reliable government sources, including MyPlate and the 2020-2025 Dietary Guidelines for Americans (DGA). This information is familiar to many people, but a refresher never hurts. Chapters 9 and 10 present ideas to improve the nutritional quality of the food at your food pantry or food kitchen. A special part of Chapter 9 is information about the SWAP nutritional ranking system. SWAP is a fantastic tool to empower clients to make informed, healthy food choices. More about SWAP can be found in Chapter 9 resources.

Cost-Effectiveness:

Whether money and resources are in abundance or shortage, most FAAs strive for cost-effectiveness. Cost efficiency allows FAAs to serve more clients. The good news is that food can be purchased and prepared affordably while maintaining remarkable quality and nutrition. Chapter 11 has tips to reduce plate cost and for planning delicious and inexpensive meals. This information is helpful for food kitchens, houses of worship, and even clients themselves. Instructions to calculate plate cost along with websites to find easy, economical recipes are linked in resources.

Chapter 4: The Organizational Assessment

The organizational assessment is a helpful resource to personally evaluate how your food assistance agency (FAA) operates. It will aid you in celebrating your strengths, identifying places to improve, and setting goals for the future. After answering these questions thoughtfully, you should have a clarified appreciation for your FAA and what aspects make it unique. Also, you should gain insight on areas where you can potentially make improvements to better meet the needs of your community.

Operation, Management, Volunteers:

These are fact-based questions that will summarize how your FAA works- the mechanics of your FAA. They provide a solid understanding of the systems, rules, and people that allow each FAA to operate. These questions provide clarity and direction for improving FAAs from a policy standpoint.

1. Are you run independently or are you overseen by another organization? Who do you answer to when making decisions for your FAA?
2. Are you partnered with a food bank?

3. Do you have regular volunteers and/or occasional volunteers?
4. How do you keep track of volunteers?
5. How do you schedule volunteers?
6. What tasks do volunteers do?
7. Overall, are you satisfied with the work your volunteers do?

Safety and Stock:

These questions are about how you obtain, store, and give away food. In addition, they clarify your collection standards- items you will and will not accept. These questions improve your understanding of the foods your FAA accepts as donatable, what they have excesses/shortages of, and how food safety is handled.

1. Where do you get donations?
2. Are there foods often in shortage or excess?
3. Do you have types of foods you do not accept?
4. How do you decide whether to keep or throw away an item you have doubts about?
5. Do you accept past-date food? At what point is it too old to keep?
6. Do you keep perishable or ready-to-eat foods?
7. Do you stock non-food items such as toiletries/sanitation products, menstrual products, kitchen supplies, etc?
8. Do you repackage foods (i.e., remove bulk items from their bag and put them in smaller bags)?

9. Do you have and regularly utilize food thermometers? What about freezer/refrigerator thermometers?
10. Overall, are you satisfied with the donations you get?
11. Overall, do you feel knowledgeable and confident about food safety?

Clients:

These questions ask about who, what, and where you provide food assistance. By answering, you learn about the demographic of clients served, identify barriers that may prevent clients from accessing your service, and understand what interactions with clients are like. Furthermore, you define how food is transferred to the client (your food distribution model).

1. What is your target demographic? Do you serve people who are food insecure, living in food deserts, displaced/homeless, etc.? Or a combination of these?
2. How many clients do you typically serve in a week? A month? A year?
3. Is there a specific geographical area you serve?
4. Do you serve the same people regularly, or do clients often come only once or twice?
5. What is your distribution method? Do you distribute standardized boxes, allow clients to

"shop" based on personal preferences, or a combination of both?

6. What specifies the type and amount of items that go in each box? Or, what items are clients limited on the amount they may take?
7. Do your clients have reliable transportation?
8. Is there a demographic you have trouble reaching?

Strengths and Challenges:

Finally, these reflective questions seek to understand how your FAA is doing on a large scale and what you want the future to be like. They provide a better understanding of how partners can come alongside your FAA and serve you as you serve others.

1. What is your FAA's greatest need?
2. Where are you thriving and where would you like to improve?
3. *Why* do you do what you do?
4. What is an actionable step that other people/agencies can take to help you?
5. Overall, are you happy with the trajectory of your FAA? If not, how would you like to improve in the future?

Chapter 5: The Barriers

Barriers may prevent potential clients from accessing and utilizing the food assistance your food assistance agency (FAA) provides. Most likely, you have identified and overcome plenty of barriers in the past. To ensure clients can easily access your services, it is essential to ask yourself one big question regularly:

What barriers, challenges, and factors prevent people who could benefit from our FAA from accessing its resources?

Here are a few more specific sub-questions you can use to identify barriers:

1. Do potential clients know about our services?
2. Do potential clients consider and feel good about utilizing our services?
3. Can potential clients obtain food at the times we offer it?
4. Can potential clients at the location we offer it?
5. Can potential clients prepare, eat, and store the food we provide?

This chapter addresses a few barriers that might exist between FAAs and clients, limiting their impact in the community. In addition, it suggests ways to eliminate these barriers.

Do potential clients know about our services?

It is not unusual for people to suddenly encounter a life crisis and be unfamiliar with the resources available in their community. It is vital that you make your FAA well known, so that when people need your service, they will think to contact you. You can (and likely already do) publicize through media, advertisements, outreach events, networking, and word-of-mouth. Maintaining a consistent presence on social media can provide information and updates to your clients. You can even spread word about other community resources your clients might utilize, such as other FAAs, programs, and community events.

Organizations like the Gateway Gaston exist to connect clients to services for which they may be unfamiliar but eligible. If you are outside of Gaston County, there may be similar organizations that can help connect clients to your services. Consider reaching out to houses of worship, community centers, and small businesses to spread awareness of your FAA.

Do potential clients consider utilizing our services?

To obtain food assistance, clients must realize they need food assistance. A potential challenge for clients is recognizing that they qualify for help.

As mentioned before, the USDA ERS has two food insecurity categories: low food security and very low food security, which used to be called "food insecurity without hunger" and "food insecurity with hunger" ("Definitions of Food Insecurity"). Clients experiencing the physical sensation of hunger will likely know that they can utilize an FAA. They will search for and access food assistance.

Clients experiencing low food security, however, have enough food to avoid physical hunger, but must sacrifice the quality or variety of their diet. For example, consider a family that eats ramen noodles for dinner every night because, by eating inexpensively, they can afford to *have* dinner every night. Clients falling into the low food security category may not realize they are food insecure, because technically, they have *enough* food. They may not recognize the benefits of accessing food assistance, or even feel guilty because they believe "other people need it more."

Recall that food *security* is "access by all people at all times to enough food for an active, healthy life" ("Food Insecurity in the U.S."). Ramen noodles have little nutritional value- they are made of refined grains, full of sodium, and lack quality protein and micronutrients. Eating ramen noodles every night does *not* support an active, healthy life. Eating them excessively to avoid hunger would compromise a person's physical health and classify them as food insecure. These clients have enough *food*, but not enough *nutrition*.

Clients in this demographic must know that food assistance is available. They must also feel good about accepting it. One way to promote this is by allowing anyone to have food and making it very clear that *anyone* can have food. Refrain from using language in publicity media like "feeding the hungry." This phrase can be humiliating, and it is inaccurate. Not everyone struggling with food insecurity experiences physical hunger. Referring to clients as "the hungry" can prevent those who are not experiencing physical hunger from accessing food assistance. It can also rob clients of their dignity.

If your FAA truly serves one exclusive demographic, such as the homeless community or children, specify that. Otherwise, using phrases such as "free vegetables" or "community meal" is more accurate, inclusive, and dignifying. After all, access and dignity are always priorities.

People experiencing low food security can unknowingly benefit from food assistance as well. FAAs do this by "masking the mission." Go into the community under the guise of providing a different service besides food assistance. For example, the Gateway is working on a mobile food pantry model, incognito as a nutrition education tent. This model pantry offers healthy eating resources, along with "healthy meal kits" that include all the ingredients to create nutrient-dense and delicious cuisine (more on meal kits in Chapter 6 and in resources under Recipes). The intent of this model is to bring nutritious food into food deserts while preserving dignity.

The model makes meal kits available to anyone and does not explicitly state that the intent is to address low food access. This increases the likelihood that people who do not identify as food insecure will take advantage of the resources. Other ideas for "masking the mission" include hosting community meals, block parties, and events, or distributing food with free fruit/vegetable stands and outdoor cupboards.

Can potential clients obtain food at the times we offer it?

When is your FAA open and serving? Hours of operation can be a barrier. If a potential client works a 9-5 job or morning shift, they cannot access your food assistance if you distribute exclusively in the morning. Similarly, if you are open only one or two days per week, people with inflexible schedules may find it challenging to visit your FAA.

There are several possible solutions. The most obvious is to expand your hours. Lengthen the time per day your FAA is open or add more days to your schedule. Opening at least one weekend day is ideal. You can also vary distribution hours. For example, if you currently distribute on Mondays, Wednesdays, Fridays, and Saturdays, you could distribute Monday mornings, Wednesday afternoons, Friday evenings, and Saturdays midday. This increases access for clients who have inflexible daily schedules.

Directors may worry about volunteer schedules when changing distribution hours. What if no one can work these new shifts? Keep in mind that like clients, volunteers have different schedules. Some may work flex-schedules, or other workweeks that deviate from the traditional 9-5. New shifts accommodate more clients, and you may gain new volunteers as well.

Can potential clients obtain food at the location we offer it?

We have discussed food deserts, and clearly, geographical location plays into food insecurity. Potential clients may know of your FAA and want to access it. However, distance or transportation issues can prevent them from receiving food. Perhaps the trip is too long, they cannot afford fuel to drive to your location, or they do not own a vehicle. (Use the USDA Food Access Research Atlas mentioned in Chapter 2 to examine how distance and vehicle ownership affects your own community. It is linked in Chapter 2 resources.)

To combat this barrier, you must get creative. One popular idea is mobile food pantries or food kitchens, which can be assembled in 18-wheeler trucks, vans, or even the trunk of a car. A collapsible tent is another option. Larger FAAs could collaborate with houses of worship or local businesses to set up and supply food to caring cupboards or small pantries, establishing a network of distribution sites. Similar approaches can be used by food kitchens. A few collapsible tables, a cooler, and a vehicle can take your food kitchen across the community, meeting clients where they are. If your FAA does not have the resources to go mobile, consider supporting a fellow FAA that is already mobile.

Can potential clients prepare, eat, and store the food we provide?

Eating and food habits are complex. Many factors influence whether the food you distribute is ultimately eaten. These barriers may prevent the food you provide from being useful.

First, clients may be unable to prepare it. Perhaps they don't have can openers, pots, a microwave, or other tools to cook it. Maybe they don't know how to use the ingredients, or don't have the cooking skills to prepare them. Clients may not eat food items because they dislike or have an allergy to them. Lastly, they could lack containers, a refrigerator, or a freezer to safely store ingredients or leftovers.

R. Dwayne Burks, Director and Chaplain of the Gateway Gaston, tells a story of how one small kitchen tool made a huge difference.

> Several years ago, a Gateway Gaston volunteer provided a Thanksgiving meal for a family in our community. After delivering the meal to the family's modest apartment

the volunteer left town for the holiday weekend.

On Thanksgiving Day, the Gateway received another request from the thankful family. You guessed it. They needed a can opener if they were going to be able to enjoy the meal together. Both family members were physically challenged and could not walk to the nearby stores. They had little or no surplus funds nor did they have a vehicle. A Gateway team member delivered a can opener Thanksgiving morning and saved the day.

A 2018 study at a food pantry in the Midwest found that many of the pantry's clients did not have access to cooking supplies. 24% had no oven, 39% had no measuring cups, and 16% lacked electricity in the kitchen (Pritt et. al. 75). Furthermore, 31% of families reported not using food they received from the pantry for some reason (Pritt et. al. 75). This study is small and localized, but it illustrates the point- you never know which resources a client can or can not access.

Perhaps the best way to beat this issue is by providing choice wherever you can. Choice provides dignity, reduces waste, and increases the cost-effectiveness of your services. Clients are free to pick food they want, are familiar and comfortable with, can prepare, and enjoy eating. Another idea is to have basic food prep/storage equipment available to distribute along with food. Can openers, forks and spoons, plastic storage boxes, and dishes are great to keep on hand.

These are a few of the numerous barriers that can affect clients of FAAs. Of course, barriers are as unique as clients themselves. The best way to combat barriers is to ask clients if anything makes utilizing your services challenging, and how you can better serve them. By regularly surveying the unique needs of your clients, you can minimize barriers or eliminate them altogether.

Chapter 6: Food Pantry Distribution Models and Mobile Pantry Sample Stock

This chapter defines and discusses different models of food distribution. Finally, a sample stock for a nutrition tent and mobile pantry is included at the conclusion.

There are many unique and wonderful FAAs in Gaston County, NC, utilizing a seemingly limitless number of distribution methods. A few examples:

1) Displaced Roses operates a mobile hot food kitchen, serving food in four different locations.
2) Bountiful Blessings distributes mass amounts of food by drive-through.
3) St. Mark's Episcopal Church provides free snacks and food items via an outdoor cupboard close to the sidewalk, which a volunteer refills daily.
4) Gaston County's crisis relief organizations (CROs) use food distribution models on a spectrum between standardized box and client-choice (discussed shortly).
5) Gastonia Street Ministry recruits houses of worship to prepare and serve meals, and

provides "blessing bags" full of food and
hygiene items.

As you can see from these examples, there are numerous ways to distribute food effectively. FAAs often provide nonperishables, snacks, or groceries in some form, and, for that reason, the focus of this chapter is placed on food pantries rather than food kitchens.

Personal observations and academic research indicate that, overall, food distribution methods commonly vary across a spectrum between two models: standardized box pantries and client-choice pantries. This chapter describes and highlights the benefits and drawbacks of these models. It also discusses how you can tweak the way you distribute food to address the needs of both your FAA and the clients you serve.

Standardized Box Distribution Model:

In a standardized box model pantry, volunteers put a standardized type and amount of food into a box and give it to the client (Thomas, Chapter 5). This may happen prior to or during distribution. The main feature of this model is that every client receives the same or similar items, and the box is assembled by someone other than the client.

The standardized box distribution model has benefits and drawbacks. The benefits are that everything is fair- clients receive the same amount of food and similar items (Thomas, Chapter 5). Clients may like the privacy of a drive-thru distribution, and many volunteers find creating and distributing standardized boxes to be fast and efficient. Pre-boxing allows food to be prepared ahead of distribution time. FAAs can easily get rid of items in excess by increasing the quantity in each box. During the COVID-19 pandemic, pre-boxing is an excellent option to reduce contact between clients and volunteers and maintain social distancing.

However, there are drawbacks to this method. Clients may find the lack of choice in what food they receive a drawback. It can rob the client of their dignity (Martin, 75). Not everyone likes having choices made for them. During a crisis, when clients already feel stressed, their food is one more part of their lives where they have no control (Martin, 73).

Additionally, the standardized box distribution model can contribute to food and resource waste (Arnold, Chapter 9). Every person and family is unique, and so dietary restrictions, personal preferences, and various other factors can result in food items going unused (Arnold, Chapter 9). Recall the mention of allergies and disliking certain foods in Chapter 5. What if a weekly pantry client dislikes beans, but always receives pinto beans in their standardized box? Similarly, perhaps the family of a child with a peanut allergy gets peanut butter every visit. Uneaten items accumulate in their pantry. Clients may re-donate them or share with a friend, but they may also allow the items to expire or discard them. Items that spoil or get discarded are ultimately a wasted resource. The client receives less usable food, and the FAA loses valuable stock.

Client-Choice Distribution Model:

In the client-choice distribution model, clients have a degree of control over the types of food they receive (Arnold, Chapter 9). This looks different for every pantry. Most have limits on what and how much of each particular item can be chosen, which ensures there is plenty of food to share (Martin, 78). For example, popular items, items in shortage, or expensive items may be limited by the FAA. Families may be directed to select one fruit and one vegetable. Government commodity food may be given to each family in a specific quantity. However, the main feature of this model is that clients ultimately have input into what groceries they take home.

The positives of client-choice are compelling. Allowing clients to choose their food drastically reduces resource waste. If the client knows their family cannot use or dislikes an item, they can simply refuse it. They can select an alternative better suited to their taste, and the FAA can give the rejected item to someone else. This increases efficiency and conserves funding and donations (Martin, 75).

The most important aspect of client-choice is the dignity it restores. Client-choice allows clients to actively participate in deciding what food they want. In many cases, client-choice pantries are designed to feel similar to shopping in a grocery store (Thomas, Chapter 5). This is reassuring to clients, and it helps them to feel comfortable, confident, and empowered. (Martin, 73-74). Dignity is always a priority.

Overall, client-choice has much support from food insecurity experts as the ideal distribution model for FAAs. However, a hybrid model may be necessary, especially in current times, as we recover from the COVID-19 pandemic. A challenge to you: introduce choice in some fashion to your regular operations. It can be as simple as allowing clients the choice between chocolate or vanilla cupcakes or asking if they prefer apples or bananas. Start small and take baby steps. Baby steps add up to huge improvements.

If, in time, you become interested in client-choice, look at these helpful resources. There is a comprehensive, step-by-step guide to converting from a standardized box model to a client-choice model from the Ohio Association of Second Harvest Food Banks called *Making the Switch: A Guide for Converting to a Client Choice Food Pantry*. It would be an excellent place to learn more.

John Arnold's *Charity Food Programs that can End Hunger in America* is an online publication with information about improving the charitable food system in your community. Jef Thomas's *How to Run A Food Pantry* is another online publication based on the best practice advice from *Charity Food Programs that can End Hunger in America*. Both of these are published on the website *End Hunger in America and* are full of wonderful reading for food pantries.

Finally, Dr. Katie S. Martin's is a thought leader in the world of charitable food systems and food insecurity, and throughout her book, <u>*Reinventing Food Banks and Pantries: New Tools to End Hunger*</u>, she advocates for client-choice and presents many wonderful strategies for improving food assistance.

All these helpful books and online publications can be accessed through links online under Further Reading in resources.

Mobile Pantry Model:

A unique distribution model is the mobile food pantry. Mobile food pantries are designed to be easily moved and distribute food in multiple locations. The strength of this model is that clients across a wide geographical area can access food assistance. This is of particular importance when addressing food deserts, where clients may live far away from affordable, healthy food.

The Gateway Gaston is designing a mobile food pantry model. It is mentioned in Chapter 5 as an example of how to "mask the mission" to reach people who do not know they can benefit from food assistance. Disguised as a "nutrition education tent," it would provide resources about healthy eating, recipes, and activities. In addition, it would distribute free healthy meal kits, with preparation instructions. The model has four meal options and would stock ten of each option at every event. On the next two pages, you will find a chart with each meal and the ingredients needed (find the printable recipe cards under Recipes in resources):

Meal Kits Sample Stock:

Meal:	Food 1	Food 2	Food 3	Food 4
Tuna Alfredo	Tuna (1-2 cans, 5 oz or larger)	Pasta, whole wheat (12oz or larger)	Alfredo (1 jar, at least 1 cup)	Peas (1 can, at least 1/2 cup)
Beans + Rice	Beans, pinto or black (1 15 oz can, at least 2 cups)	Rice, brown, (at least 4 cup prepared, 1 cup dry)	Salsa (1 jar, any size)	Corn (1 can, at least 1 cup)
PBJ Wraps	Peanut butter, natural if possible (1 jar, any size) (at least 8 tbs)	Jelly, sugar free if possible (1 jar, any size) (at least 8 tbs)	Tortillas, whole wheat (at least 4 tortillas, 8" or larger)	Fruit cups/appl esauce (4)
Peanut Butter Oatmeal	Oats, plain (not flavored), (8 instant packets or 18 oz or larger)	Peanut butter, natural if possible (1 jar, any size) (at least 8 tbs)	Cinnamo n or cocoa powder (1, any size)	Fruit cups (4) or raisins boxes (4)

Based on a goal of bringing 10 of each of these meals per outing, here is the stock that would be necessary:

- 10-20 cans of tuna, 5 oz or larger
- 10-20 cans beans, 15oz (at least 2 cups)
- 20 jars peanut butter, any size (at least 8 tbs)
- 10 containers of rice, brown, enough to have 4+ cups prepared (about 1 cup dry)
- 10 12oz+ containers of pasta, 12oz or larger, whole grain
- 10 8+ instant pack boxes or 10 tub of oats 18oz or larger, whole grain
- 10 cans of corn, 15oz (at least 1 cup)
- 10 packs of tortillas, 4+ per bag, 8" or larger, whole grain
- 10 cans peas, 15oz or smaller (at least 1/2 cup)
- 80 Fruit cups/applesauce, or 40 fruit cups and 40 boxes of raisins
- 10 jars sugar free jelly, any size (at least 4 tbs)
- 10 jars salsa, any size
- 10 jars alfredo, 16oz (at least 2 cups)
- 10 containers cinnamon or cocoa powder, any size

Purchase items in light, easy to open packaging, and opt for pre-cooked whenever you can. For example, buy cans with pop-cap lids that do not require a can opener, or prepared rather than dry rice. Avoid putting several heavy items in one bag. This ensures that children, the elderly, and homeless recipients can easily use the meal kits.

The amount of stock can be adjusted based on the number of meal kits distributed in the first few weeks of operation, which kits are the most popular, and feedback from the visitors of the mobile pantry/nutrition tent. We hope that this model proves useful to increase food access in local food deserts.

Chapter 7: The Basics of Food Safety

Food must be safe before anything else. Without food safety procedures, productive food assistance cannot be done. Lives cannot be improved because clients are at constant risk of becoming sick. Food safety often seems like common sense, but it is more complex than many realize. However, once you have the knowledge required to obtain, store, handle, and prepare food safely, you can confidently prevent foodborne illness.

The Centers for Disease Control and Prevention estimates that one in six Americans becomes sick from foodborne pathogens or contaminants each year, around 128,000 are hospitalized, and 3,000 die ("Burden of Foodborne Illness: Findings.") Clients of food assistance agencies (FAAs) are often affected by chronic disease (the reasons are discussed in Chapter 8). The Hunger in America 2014 Study was prepared for Feeding America, and it reports these important survey data points that illustrate why clients can be especially vulnerable to foodborne illnesses:

- 58% of surveyed client households have a member with high blood pressure (Weinfeld et. al. 119)

- 33% have a member with diabetes (Weinfeld et. al. 119).
- 28.6% of households have no health insurance (Weinfeld et. al. 121)
- 55.1% had unpaid medical bills (Weinfeld et. al. 121)

This data demonstrates that clients of FAAs have a high rate of chronic disease, and a low ability to access health and emergency care. Thus, it is imperative to maintain food safety in FAAs for the health and well-being of clients.

A quick disclaimer- this chapter is hand-picked information that is important to FAAs, especially small FAAs that provide groceries or cook for small groups of clients. Please *don't consider this a comprehensive guide to food safety*. One chapter of a book cannot comprehensively encompass everything you should know.

Investing in a food safety training certification can provide a solid understanding of food safety. Have at least one director, staff member, or key volunteer certified. ServSafe's Food Handler course is excellent. ServSafe offers courses for specific audiences, such as managers, and on specific topics, such as allergen safety. The courses are also very affordable. A link to ServSafe can be found under Chapter 7 in resources.

This chapter covers four main areas where food safety can be controlled in an FAA, in chronological order: stock safety, storage safety, personal hygiene, and preparation safety. By understanding how to control food safety from purchase to service, you can do your part to keep clients safe from foodborne illness.

Stock Safety:

The stock you purchase or receive is the starting point of food safety, and the foundation of everything going forward. The stock you cook with and/or distribute must be stored safely.

A common point of confusion for consumers is product dating. According to the USDA Food Safety and Inspection Service (FSIS), most food products have a date on the package that indicates when to use it ("Food Product Dating"). However, food producers are not legally required to date their products (except for baby formula, which must maintain peak quality and nutrients). ("Food Product Dating").

Two aspects of food product dating produce the most uncertainty for consumers. Firstly, the terms used to label products can be inconsistent. The FSIS recommends that producers use "Best if Used By" to avoid confusing consumers; however, others like "Sell By," "Use By," and "Freeze By" dates are also common ("Food Product Dating"). These terms have different meanings. This table summarizes those explained online by the FSIS in their "Food Product Dating" article:

Glossary of Food Dates:

"Best if Used By"	The product is of best *quality* if used before or around this date. It can be safely consumed after this date, but may not be at peak flavor or texture.
"Sell By"	Retail stores should not sell the product after this date, because its quality is likely to go down. The product can still be safely consumed after this date.
"Use By"	The final date the product is at peak quality. It can be used after this date, but the quality may be reduced. *The exception is baby formula.* Baby formula should not be used after this date.
"Freeze By"	The product should be frozen by this date to keep it at peak quality.

FoodSafety.gov has a helpful resource for keeping quality high when storing food. The Foodkeeper App informs consumers about how to store a variety of items, as well as how long they can be stored in the pantry, refrigerator, or freezer at peak quality. It is a useful tool for FAAs and can be found online or as an app for mobile devices. It is linked in Chapter 7 resources.

To introduce the second point, please note the word *quality* in every definition. Unfortunately, confusion regarding these dates can result in unnecessary food waste.

Best practice is to *always* use common sense and your five senses. According to the USDA FSIS's article "Food Product Dating," as long as food has been properly handled, it should be safe to consume. Make sure food does not show noticeable signs of spoilage (mold, foul smell, milky liquid, etc.) and has been properly handled at all times. If a food looks or smells less than optimal, or has been stored or handled unsafely, throw it away ("Food Product Dating"). Prevent spoilage by practicing FIFO (first in, first out- use the oldest food first) and by checking the quality of your food regularly. By doing this, you can reduce food and resource waste while maintaining food safety.

Spoiled food may be obviously spoiled, but sometimes it is tricky to spot. When purchasing salvage food, taking donations, or inspecting current stock, watch for the following signs that the U.S. Food and Drug Administration (FDA) considers indicative of unsafe food ("Surplus, Salvaged, and Donated Foods"):

- Are cans swollen, bulging, dented, leaking, or poorly sealed?
    - Swollen or bulging cans may have bacteria growing inside.
    - Cans or packages that are heavily dented, leaking, torn, or poorly sealed may have been exposed to bacteria.
- Has the food been maintained at its proper temperature?
    - Ensure food has been stored as intended. Refrigerated items need to have stayed refrigerated, frozen items should be still frozen.
- Has it been thawed and refrozen? Is it frostbitten, covered in ice crystals, or frozen into one lump?
    - These signs point towards improper handling, which can reduce the frozen item's quality and safety.
- Have the labels or packaging been changed?
    - It is vital you have accurate information about the food's identity, age, and ingredients. This allows you to be aware of any allergens or recalls.
- Does the package appear to have been repackaged or resealed?

- Repackaging and resealing food expose them to the environment and allow bacteria to grow.

Many FAAs feel uncomfortable distributing past-date food, especially those with less control over how food was handled before it was donated. For other FAAs, distributing past-date food is a wise use of resources. Pick the one with which you are most comfortable.

Regularly checking stock for food recalls is similarly important. Food recalls occur anytime a product is believed to be a hazard to public health ("Recalls and Outbreaks"). Possible reasons for a recall are bacterial, foreign object, or chemical contamination, as well as allergens that are incorrectly labeled ("Recalls and Outbreaks"). Recalled items should be returned to the store for a refund or discarded in order to protect consumers.

FAAs need to regularly check for U.S. Food and Drug Administration (FDA) recalls ensuring the recalled products are not present in their stock. An up-to-date list of publicized recalls is posted on the FDA website (find the webpage in Chapter 7 resources). You can also subscribe and have them delivered to your email inbox.

Properly handling stock is the first step towards preventing foodborne illness and keeping clients healthy. Next, stock must be properly stored.

Storage Safety:

The temperature at which you store shelf-stable food influences the speed that its quality deteriorates. Store all canned and shelf-stable goods in a cool, dry location, such as a pantry. Do not store food outdoors, or in an uncontrolled environment for long periods of time. The risk of quality degrading drastically increases when shelf-stable goods are stored in temperature extremes ("Shelf-Stable Food Safety").

Dr. Beverley Hammond is a Registered Dietitian and retired Carson-Newman University faculty member. She taught classes in food preparation and foodservice for many years and has ample experience in foodservice and food safety. Dr. Hammond says it is ideal that shelf stable food is stored at least six inches off the floor and away from walls. This prevents dirt, pests, water, and other contaminants from ruining stock.

> "Food needs to be kept off the floor to keep pests, dirt and water away. Also, if there is a water leak and floods the storeroom, it will probably not be six inches high. You don't want bugs and mice climbing up the wall then jumping on the food."

At the Greater Gaston Baptist Association, shelf-stable food is stored on shelves with wheels. Not only does this keep food off the floor and away from walls, but the pantry can also be easily rearranged. Shelves can be moved into a corner to make room for a meeting or event, allowing the space to be multi-purpose. In addition, floors can be easily and thoroughly cleaned.

Refrigerated, frozen, and fresh goods are wonderful to distribute. Nutritious foods like fruits, vegetables, dairy, and meat can be preserved in a refrigerator or freezer. Key steps must be taken to store these items safely. Keep food out of the "temperature danger zone." The temperature danger zone is anywhere between 40° F-140° F. When food stays between 40° F-140° F, bacteria can multiply quickly and make the food unsafe ("4 Steps to Food Safety"). Keep hot foods *very hot* and cold foods *very cold* at all times.

Keep a thermometer in the refrigerator and freezer. Make sure the refrigerators and freezers are being checked regularly and kept consistently at or below the correct temperature. Refrigerators should be 40° F or lower, and freezers should be set to 0° F or lower ("4 Steps to Food Safety"). Appliance thermometers are fairly inexpensive and easy to use, and they help you keep your refrigerators and freezers doing their job efficiently, safely, and consistently ("Are You Storing Food Safely?").

Personal Hygiene Safety:

Without volunteers and staff, FAAs could not distribute as much food, prepare as many meals, and improve so many lives. Workers are critical for the operation of FAAs, so the personal hygiene, attire, and actions of workers are critical for food safety. Keep policies in place allowing workers to play a role in food safety.

When discussing personal hygiene and food safety, the obvious first thought is handwashing. Everyone knows the importance of washing their hands, especially while preparing food. Wash your hands before, during, and after preparing food ("Kitchen Handwashing"). Also wash your hands after visiting the restroom, after handling uncooked foods such as meats and eggs, after using cleaning supplies, after touching your face, body, or hair, and after coughing or sneezing ("Kitchen Handwashing").

A 2015 study examined the operating procedures of 105 North Carolina food pantries. During this study, researchers observed handwashing in only 13 pantries (Chaifetz and Chapman, 2039). Handwashing when handling packaged or shelf-stable goods is less critical than handwashing before touching unpackaged foods. However, it is a fast action with the potential to prevent clients from getting sick. Frequent handwashing should be implemented with any type of food handling.

It is equally important that workers be safely and hygienically dressed. Dr. Beverley Hammond always instructs students to dress safely and hygienically while in the kitchen. In a personal interview, she explains why wearing hair restraints, keeping hands clean and polish-free, and removing jewelry are important when preparing food.

> "In addition to personal hygiene, attention should be paid to hair, nails and jewelry. Hair restraints are required around food because hair can have dirt and oil. To prevent hair getting into food, hair restraints are a must. If hair is long, it should be tied back before a hat is put on to prevent hair hanging over the shoulders and over the food. Beard protectors are also required for the same reason hair restraints are necessary. Hair getting into the food must be prevented."

Dr. Hammond points out that nail polish can be unhygienic as well.

> "During food handling, clean hands are a must. They should be free of dirt and nail polish which can chip off and get into the food. Nail polish can hide dirt under the fingernails." Clearly,

nail polish can be unsafe for the person who eats your food because it can result in food becoming contaminated. "In order to make certain nails are clean, they should be scrubbed with a fingernail brush before food handling is done."

Jewelry is also hazardous in the kitchen.

"Not only is jewelry a source of dirt which can get into food, it is a safety hazard as well. Necklaces, dangling earrings and rings on fingers can get caught on or in food production equipment causing serious injury. Jewelry should be limited to wedding rings. When handling food, gloves should be worn which will protect food from contamination."

Lastly, Dr. Hammond details what proper kitchen attire looks like and why it is important to wear disposable gloves.

"Clean, modest clothing and close-toed shoes are a must. Disposable gloves should be worn and changed frequently. Gloves are especially important if a worker has false nails or nail polish on, because if it chips, it could get into the food and contaminate it."

Preparation Safety:

FAAs serving prepared meals know how complex yet vital it is to maintain food safety in the kitchen. Environmental elements must be controlled in a food kitchen to prevent foodborne illness.

Cross-contamination is when different foods come into contact with each other, introducing pathogens to a previously safe food ("What is Cross Contamination?". This often occurs when foods like meat, poultry, seafood, or eggs are prepared near other foods, on the same surface, or using the same utensils ("What is Cross Contamination?"). Ensure cooking equipment is sanitized after preparing these foods- Better yet, use separate equipment. Change your gloves and wash your hands thoroughly between handling different foods ("4 Steps to Food Safety").

Once everything is chopped, sliced, peeled, and prepared, it is time to start cooking. How cooked is cooked enough? There are a few guidelines to follow, particularly when cooking meats, poultry, seafood, and eggs.

Each of these animal-based foods must reach a minimum internal temperature before they are safe to eat. These range from 145° F-165° F and vary depending on the food being cooked ("Safe Minimum Internal Temperature Chart"). The best way to measure internal temperature is by using a food thermometer ("Safe Minimum Internal Temperature Chart"). Thermometers are affordable and easy to use. A helpful safe internal temperature chart from the FSIS is linked in Chapter 7 resources.

Leftovers may be stored in the refrigerator or frozen for future use. Ensure the refrigerator is 40° F or less, and if refrigerating large quantities of food, divide it into multiple containers or pieces so the whole food cools quickly ("Refrigeration & Food Safety"). If it cools too slowly, the food might remain in the temperature danger zone for an extended period of time.

In conclusion, food safety is critical for the wellbeing of clients, volunteers, and the community. Not only do these standards prevent foodborne illnesses, but they also convey to clients that their health and safety is valued by the FAA serving them. Always set food safety standards and adhere to them, so that you can make a safe and positive impact on the clients you serve. Food safety standards maintain health, wellness, and dignity.

Chapter 8: The Basics of Nutrition

Nutrition is defined by the Merriam-Webster English Dictionary as "the act or process of nourishing or being nourished, *specifically*: the sum of the processes by which an animal or plant takes in and utilizes food substances." Good nutrition is essential. Eating healthy provides the nutrients and fuel we need to live long, healthy, and fulfilling lives. It increases energy, aids in maintaining a healthy weight, and helps children to grow and develop properly. Eating healthy reduces the chance of developing chronic diseases, such as type 2 diabetes, cardiovascular disease, high blood pressure, and cancer. Good nutrition is the foundation of good health, and health is the foundation of a happy life.

Despite all the benefits, eating healthy is a struggle. Any honest person admits that it requires exceptional willpower to eat an apple instead of a cookie. While it is unrealistic and unnecessary to eat perfectly every day, maintaining an overall healthy diet is necessary. However, the challenge is often greater for those dealing with food insecurity. This chapter examines the link between food insecurity and chronic disease, outlines basic nutrition information, and describes the food groups based on MyPlate and the 2020-2025 Dietary Guidelines for Americans.

Health and Nutrition Implications of Food Insecurity:

People struggling with food insecurity face challenges that make healthy eating difficult, and they have real consequences. A large and often cited 2016 study using data from a variety of sources shows that food insecurity is associated with much higher-than-average healthcare expenses (Berkowitz et. al). This data is visualized by the Feeding America Research team in an interactive graphic linked in Chapter 8 resources. Using this graphic, you can access data for any state and county in the United States.

According to this Feeding America graphic, in Gaston County, it is estimated that food-insecure individuals spend roughly $1,740 more annually to cover medical expenses than their food-secure neighbors (Feeding America Research). Nationally, this is estimated to have totaled in 2016 to approximately *$52.9 billion dollars* in excess healthcare costs (Feeding America Research).

A 2010 article by Seligman and Shillinger describes a cyclic model of how food insecurity and chronic disease exacerbate one another. Food insecurity causes people to use "coping strategies" like eating more inexpensive, nutrient-poor foods. Overall poor health is the result due to the link between diet and chronic diseases such as diabetes, hypertension, and obesity. Having a chronic disease increases medical costs and may negatively impact job opportunities, causing budget strain and further hurting the person's ability to afford healthy food. Plus, the constant stress of food insecurity negatively affects health and disease management throughout the cycle (Seligman & Shillinger). A graphical depiction of this concept, illustrated by Feeding America, is available on their Hunger and Health website (which you can find under Chapter 8 resources).

Food truly is medicine, and, like medicine, not everyone can afford it. Our healthcare system is broken, and so is our food system. What can be done?

What Can Be Done?

How can you help? You are already helping to improve the health of your community by running a food assistance agency (FAA). Supplementary food, no matter how healthful, does wonders for the stress levels of your neighbors, thereby improving quality of life. However, the nutritional quality of the food you provide matters, too, especially for preventing chronic disease. Look to Chapters 9 and

10 for tips about improving nutrition in food pantries and food kitchens.

Basic Nutrition:

Food and nutrition information is everywhere, but unfortunately, so is misinformation. For every internet article touting a "superfood" another calls the same food "toxic." Search "is (insert any food) bad for you" on the internet, and with some digging, you can find at least one article demonizing that food. Same with diets- people will insist that their favorite (keto, plant-based, paleo, raw vegan, intermittent fasting, etc.) is the sole road to true health. Because it is difficult to get reliable nutrition information, only U.S. government resources and peer-reviewed journal articles are referenced in this chapter. Particularly, the 2020-2025 Dietary Guidelines for Americans (DGA) is an important source.

There are two ways to think about nutrition and categorize food. They are complementary, but different. The first way is food groups. This method is helpful because it is a straightforward, easy way to emphasize the importance of a rich, varied diet. Think of the MyPlate graphic from MyPlate:

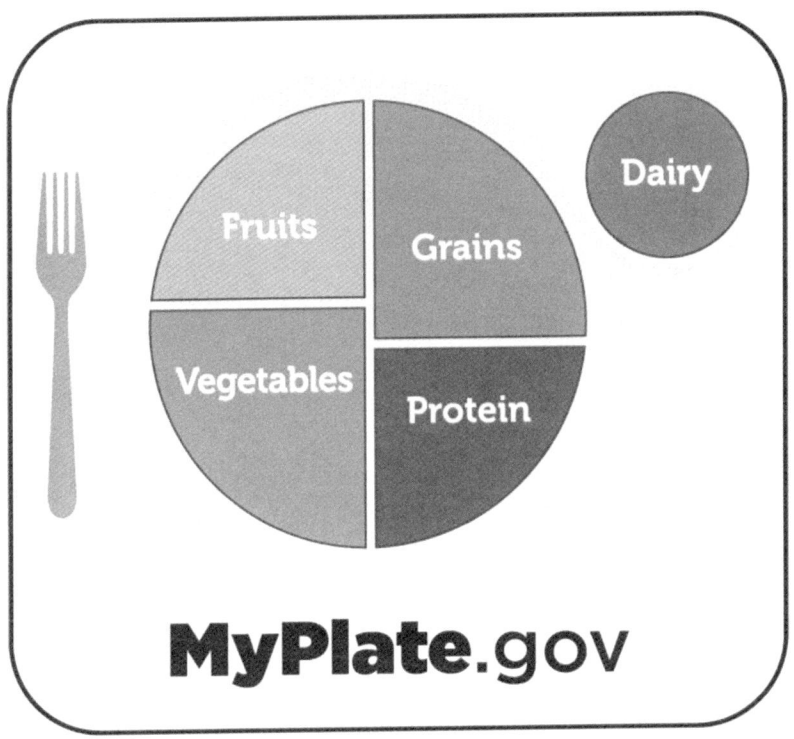

Image used with permission from the USDA, retrieved from MyPlate.gov

The 2020-2025 DGA and MyPlate (the most current government-endorsed nutrition resources) both describe nutrition primarily with food groups. The beauty of food groups is that they are user-friendly, colorful, and visual. They provide a framework rather than exact nutrient requirements, encouraging healthy and diverse dietary patterns no matter what foods you prefer (DGA, 6). Food groups also allow people of varying ages and cultures to customize their plates according to personal preference and which foods they find culturally acceptable (DGA, 6).

The second way to think about nutrition is macronutrients and micronutrients. This method is more scientific, explaining the physical molecules that make up food, like carbohydrates, proteins, fats, vitamins, minerals, and water. Learning how the human body uses nutrients provides a factual, quantitative understanding of nutrition. Unfortunately, macronutrients and micronutrients are complex, and ultimately beyond the scope of this chapter because of the detail required to fully understand them. Resources for anyone curious about the science of nutrition are provided in Chapter 8 resources.

The most important thing to know is that a healthy diet requires eating a variety of foods. Employing food groups when working in an FAA is an easy and fun way to promote this dietary variety.

Food Groups:

This section explains the concept of food groups and how foods are categorized to help consumers eat a nutritionally adequate diet. MyPlate.gov, a United States government website that provides educational resources based on the Dietary Guidelines for Americans (DGA), sorts foods into five major groups:

1) Vegetables
2) Fruits
3) Grains
4) Proteins
5) Dairy/fortified soy alternatives

Here is the graphic again. It shows the proportions of each food group that make up a healthy diet in a visually pleasing format:

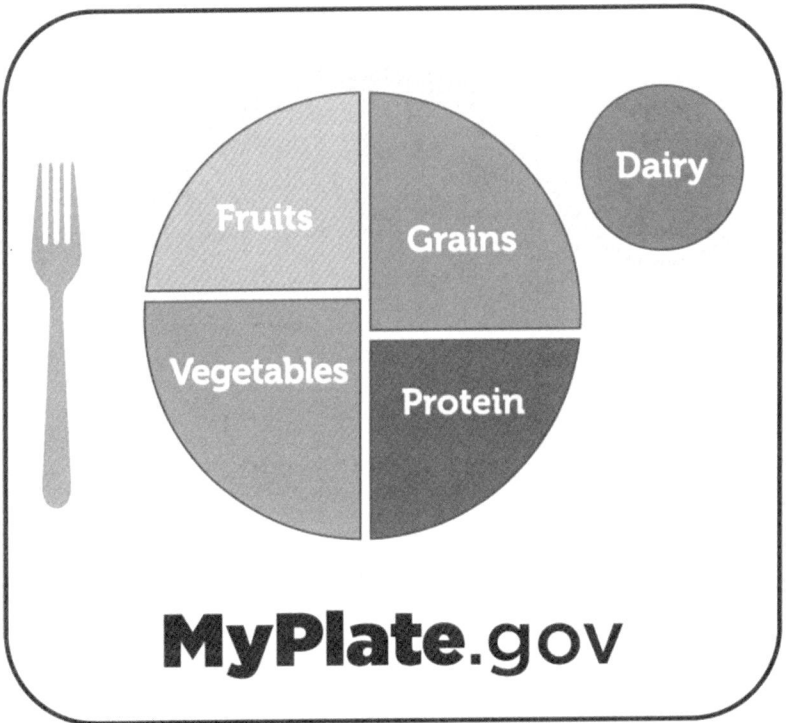

Image used with permission from the USDA, retrieved from MyPlate.gov

The DGA suggests that we increase our consumption of fruits, vegetables, whole grains, low-fat dairy products, seafood, and beans/peas/lentils (DGA, 31-34). In addition, we should limit added sugars, saturated fats, sodium, and alcoholic beverages to 15% or less of our total calorie intake (DGA, 37).

The DGA recommends this amount from each food group in a 2,000-calorie diet (DGA, Appendix 3):
- 2 cups of fruit
- 2 1/2 cups of vegetables
- 6 ounces of grains (equal to 3 cups rice or 6 slices of bread)
- 5 1/2 ounces protein foods (roughly equal to 6 eggs, 1 can of tuna, or 1 1/2 cups of beans)
- 3 cups of dairy foods

Food group guidelines for other calorie levels are different and can be found in either Appendix 3 of the DGA or on the MyPlate website. A quiz on MyPlate.gov is available to determine your own calorie level based on height, weight, age, and physical activity level. By following these guidelines, we can maximize our nutrition and health benefits and maintain dietary balance. Upcoming is a more detailed description of each food group, and explanations of unique or "other" foods not explicitly included in a food group.

Vegetables:

Eating plenty of vegetables is vital to health. Vegetables provide dietary fiber and tons of micronutrients. The 2020-2025 DGA says there are five subtypes of vegetables: dark green, red/orange, beans/peas/lentils (more about their classification later), starchy, and other vegetables (DGA, 31). Eat a variety of all of these vegetable subtypes, because each one has unique micronutrients that are essential to health (DGA, 31).

Fruits:

Fruit is delicious and nutritious due to its sweetness and high nutrient-density. It is a source of energizing simple carbohydrates, fiber, and micronutrients, and should be a consistent part of every diet. The DGA says that fresh, canned, and dried fruits count towards fruit intake. Be mindful of added sugar. 100% fruit juice counts towards fruit intake as well, but most of the fruit we eat should be from whole, unprocessed fruits. (DGA, 32).

Grains:

Grains make up a large portion of our diet. Grains are often found in mixed dishes, such as casserole, stir-fry, pizza, and cookies. Always make half of your grains whole, and limit white, refined grains. Whole-grain options are not always available for mixed dishes. Choose whole grains when you can, and eat healthy sources, limiting foods such as cookies and cakes that contain added sugars, butter, and salt (DGA, 32-33).

Protein Foods:
Protein foods are essential to well-being. Proteins are the building blocks of many elements of the human body, such as tissues, enzymes, hormones, and blood ("Protein Foods"). Protein is found in many foods, such as meat, poultry, seafood, nuts/seeds, and eggs. Foods from other groups, such as beans/peas/lentils and dairy, contain protein too. Use leaner (low-fat) proteins such as chicken, and include oily seafood for healthy fats (DGA, 33).

Dairy/Fortified Soy Alternatives:
Dairy contains vitamin D, calcium, vitamin B12, and other important minerals for building strong bones. It is also a valuable source of protein, especially for vegetarians. The healthiest dairy is fat-free or low-fat dairy ("Dairy").

According to the DGA, people who do not consume dairy products (possible reasons include having a milk allergy, lactose intolerance, being vegan, or personal preference), can count soy alternatives as part of the dairy food group (DGA, 33). However, alternatives made with almond, hemp, coconut, or others do not count, since their nutrients are not similar to dairy (DGA, 33).

Others:

Other foods not depicted in the MyPlate graphic but discussed in the 2020-2025 DGA are oils and beverages. Because these are necessary for a healthy and varied diet, they must be mentioned. Lastly, beans, peas, and lentils are classified as "unique foods" and are beneficial in the diet.

Oils and fats are an important element of the diet in very small amounts, because they provide healthy fats. MyPlate suggests that consumers choose vegetable-based oils that are liquid at room temperature. Animal-based oils, coconut oil, and palm oil are solid at room temperature and tend to be less healthy due to higher levels of saturated fat. In general, healthy fats are liquid at room temperature while saturated fats are solid and less healthy ("More Key Topics"). Other great sources of oils are nuts, olives, fatty fish, and avocado ("More Key Topics").

Beverages are also a source of nutrients. Generally, the best option is always water. However, other choices, such as calorie-free drinks and nutritious beverages like milk and 100% fruit juice, can improve health and contribute to nutrient requirements. Also consider coffee and tea that is low in sugars and fats (DGA, 35).

The DGA calls beans, peas, and lentils "unique foods" because they fit into a category of vegetables called "pulses." They can be counted towards the vegetable group or the protein foods group ("Beans, Peas, and Lentils").

Chapter 9: Nutrition in a Food Pantry

As mentioned before, healthy food can be inaccessible for those struggling with food insecurity and/or living in food deserts. Geographical location and cost are barriers to healthy eating. For that reason, food pantries serve a major role in food and nutritional justice for communities.

Many food banks and pantries emphasize making fresh, healthy foods available to their clients. This chapter presents several ideas to increase the amount of nutritious foods given to or selected by clients. In addition, it discusses SWAP, a system used for ranking the healthfulness of foods so that nutritious items can be promoted to clients.

Standardized Box Method:

Pantries using a standardized box distribution method often use an outline that specifies what items go in each box. For some, this outline may simply describe what government commodity food is required to go in each box, while others have more detailed frameworks. Outlines allow you to control your stock while also ensuring clients receive a variety of foods from all food groups. Here are some ideas using an outline to assemble standardized boxes that include plenty of nutritious food.

MyPlate-Balanced Boxes:

Making boxes that resemble MyPlate ensures that clients receive a balanced array of different foods. Many FAAs already focus on balance, and this helps clients to meet nutrient requirements and maintain a healthy diet. To refresh, the 2020-2025 Dietary Guidelines for Americans (DGA) recommends these amounts of each food group for a 2,000-calorie diet (DGA, Appendix 3):

- 2 cups of fruits
- 2 1/2 cups of vegetables
- 6 ounces of grains (equal to 3 cups rice or 6 slices of bread)
- 5 1/2 ounces protein foods (roughly equal to 6 eggs, 1 can of tuna, 1 1/2 cups of beans)
- 3 cups of dairy foods

For simplicity, focus on achieving a good balance and representing every food group in your standardized boxes. No need to overcomplicate, just make sure each box has equal proportions of fruits, vegetables, grains, protein foods, and dairy foods. The important thing is to provide foods from every food group, so clients can eat a healthy, balanced diet.

Meal Kits:

As discussed in Chapter 6, a barrier clients may face is the inability to cook with the items they receive from a food pantry. Here is an illustrative story to demonstrate what this barrier might look like.

Dan visits a food pantry and is excited to see what is inside his box. The first two items are taco seasoning and pasta sauce. Dan realizes he has no pasta for spaghetti, nor does he have tortillas or beans for tacos. Next is a pack of deli lunch meat. Dan's refrigerator is old and works poorly. The meat may spoil if stored inside this refrigerator, so he decides he will eat a sandwich for lunch soon. Next, Dan grabs a jar of peanut butter and quickly discards it because he is allergic to peanuts. The next jar is full of olives. Dan dislikes the taste and texture of olives. The last item is a bag of dry rice. Dan loves rice but is not good at preparing it. His rice always turns out too soggy. Disappointed, Dan sets several items aside to donate back to the food pantry and makes himself a sandwich.

When given a standardized box, clients may get assorted, mismatched items, or items they dislike. Remember that everyone has unique personal preferences, dietary needs, likes, dislikes, habits, and other factors that affect what they eat. Culture and ethnic background play into food choices. In addition, food, much like slang, fashion, and music, goes in and out of style. The tastes of each generation can be drastically different. For example, an older person may prefer foods like pasta salad, saltine crackers, and roast beef, while a young adult is interested in sushi and veggie burgers.

Notice the client demographic you serve and match the food you distribute to their preferences to the best of your ability. Pay attention to client feedback and note any items that are frequently returned to your pantry. Consider surveying clients to learn what foods they enjoy receiving, and what foods they do not use.

Clients also may not have cooking tools to prepare the ingredients- they may lack a quality stove, refrigerator, can opener, or pots (Pritt et. al.). Additionally, they may not know how to cook meals with ingredients they get. If a client receives beans but no rice or tortillas, they may not eat the beans.

One simple way to address these two issues is by assembling meal kits. You may already do this without realizing. For example, maybe volunteers add tomato sauce to a standardized box with pasta or include a jar of jelly with every jar of peanut butter. Meal kits are a practical and fun way to reduce food waste after distribution. It allows clients to try new things and empowers them to build confidence in the kitchen. Meal kits are versatile, and easy for volunteers to create.

Here are a few meal kit ideas, made with 5 or fewer shelf-stable ingredients:
1) Tuna Alfredo Pasta: Pasta, alfredo sauce, canned tuna, and canned peas
2) Beans & Rice: Brown rice, canned beans, salsa, canned corn
3) PB&J Wraps: Tortillas, peanut butter, jelly, and fruit
4) Peanut Butter Oatmeal: Oats, peanut butter, and toppings

Some require basic cooking equipment, like a microwave or stove, and others, like the PB&J wraps, require only a plate and utensils. Create other options using your available shelf-stable, fresh, and frozen ingredients. Think spaghetti, burritos, vegetable soup, chicken stir fry, beef stew, and so on. You can assemble meal kits with foods you have in excess to help balance out stock. Or try incorporating popular, novel, or unfamiliar foods so clients can try an exciting new dish.

Always include instructions for meal kit preparation. Recipe handouts for the prior examples are included in the Recipe resources section of this book. Preparation might look self-explanatory, but instructions never hurt. Some clients may be new to cooking or have children helping prepare meals for the family. It is hard to know how much cooking knowledge someone has.

Client-Choice Method:

FAAs that use a primarily client-choice distribution method may also utilize an outline. The purpose in this case is to direct clients on what food they should choose. Your biggest nutrition-related challenge may be helping clients select more healthy foods. Clients likely want to eat healthy. But they may be unfamiliar with the healthy foods in stock, find preparing them daunting, or have special dietary needs to maintain a chronic medical condition. For many, it is challenging to choose the best food for their personal health needs in a food pantry.

An interesting solution is a nutrition ranking system. Nutrition ranking systems use specific nutrients to categorize foods by degree of healthfulness. There are several ranking systems that have been specifically designed for food pantries over the years, such as Feeding America's Detailed Foods to Encourage (F2E), the Nutrient Rich Foods system (NRF), Choose Healthy Options System (CHOP), and Supporting Wellness At Pantries (SWAP). (Martin et. al., 554).

SWAP was developed by Dr. Katie S. Martin, a recognized thought leader on food security and the Executive Director of the Foodshare Institute for Hunger Research and Solutions (Martin, "About the Author"). The purpose of SWAP is to increase the supply and demand for healthy food in food pantries (Martin et. al., 554).

SWAP assigns a food one of three colors: green, yellow, or red. Green foods are the healthiest, and foods to "choose often." Yellow is "choose sometimes" and red is "choose rarely" (Martin, 106). The colors resemble a stoplight, making them understandable for anyone speaking languages besides English, or with limited literacy skills (Martin, 106). Rankings align with the Dietary Guidelines for Americans (DGA) because they are based on saturated fat, sodium, and sugar levels (Martin, 106). The DGA says that these three nutrients contribute the most to chronic disease (DGA, 37).

SWAP is wonderful because it is three-tiered, including a category of "sometimes foods." Simple guidelines for ranking foods make the system volunteer-friendly. SWAP can be used to both support healthy choices for clients and request healthier items from donors (Martin, 106). Overall, SWAP is a fantastic tool for any client-choice pantry, whether implemented entirely or only partially. SWAP is free to use in any pantry. Posters, signs, labels, and informational materials are available for purchase. If you are interested in SWAP, a toolkit with further information is linked in Chapter 9 resources. You can also learn more by reading Dr. Martin's book, _Reinventing Food Banks and Pantries : New Tools to End Hunger._

Chapter 10: Nutrition in a Food Kitchen

Meals served at your food kitchen can make a huge difference in the overall quality of a client's diet and health. Good nutrition in food kitchens is impactful. By making small menu changes and swapping ingredients for nutrient-dense alternatives, you can drastically improve your meals without impacting taste, quality, or cost. Here are suggestions for nutrition in food kitchens.

The best tip is to emulate the MyPlate graphic as much as possible. Incorporate whole grains, proteins, dairy, fruits, and a sizable amount of vegetables into every meal. Perfection is not the goal, but variety is key. If meals are prepared by outside volunteers, consider creating a "plate template" or other guidelines that specify what you want included in each meal. Of course, keep it simple and lenient. For example, suggest that volunteers include one vegetable when cooking, or request that water be a beverage option at every meal.

Also be mindful of ingredients. Pay attention to the added sugar, sodium, and saturated fat on the label. Make swaps if necessary. For example, if you serve canned peaches with cream for dessert, consider buying peaches canned in 100% juice or labeled "no added sugar." You could buy low-fat or sugar-free whipped cream topping. Similarly, try seasoning meat with lemon or lime juice instead of marinades high in salt. Below are additional ideas for menu and ingredient swaps.

Menu Change Ideas:

1) **Include a fruit or vegetable** as a side dish at every meal.
2) **Plan meals that incorporate vegetables.** For example, add steamed broccoli to pasta, or extra carrots and celery to chicken noodle soup. You could even try zucchini bread or black bean brownies (if you are feeling particularly adventurous).
3) **Experiment with new ways to cook vegetables.** Roasting, adding new seasonings, or using a small amount of cheese or sauce makes vegetables more enjoyable.
4) **Choose lean, minimally processed meats.** Use canned tuna, chicken, and turkey more often than ground beef, hot dogs, lunch meat, and sausages.
5) **Minimize oil.** Try streaming, brazing, boiling, and baking as alternatives to frying.
6) **Vary your seasonings to reduce sodium content.** Common culprits of hidden sodium

are canned and processed foods, seasonings, and condiments. Salt-free seasoning blends, lemons and limes, red pepper, and garlic are a few low-sodium options. It is unnecessary and unrealistic to cut all salty seasonings but switching things up occasionally can make a big difference in controlling sodium.

7) **Use portion-controlled desserts.** Examples are gelatin, puddings, fun-size candy, single-serving prepackaged cookies and cakes, and fruit topped with whipped cream.

Ingredient Swap Ideas:

1) **Replace chips or pretzels** with **dried fruit, dried vegetables, or nuts** as snacks.

2) Use fruit juice, dried fruit, and canned fruit that says **"100% juice", or "no added sugar."**

3) Occasionally **swap starchy vegetables** like potatoes and green peas for other vegetables.

4) **Use fruit in its whole form** as often as possible.

5) **Switch white bread to whole-wheat bread** or try whole-wheat tortillas for variety.

6) **Use whole-wheat pasta** and mix vegetables into the pasta for bulk.

7) **Use Greek yogurt** in place of sour cream.

8) **Switch to skim or low-fat** dairy products.
9) **Purchase any low-sodium options** you find. Canned or processed foods, lunch meat, soups, condiments, and snack foods are often high in sodium, but low sodium versions may be available. Also, some canned foods like beans or vegetables can be rinsed to reduce sodium.
10) **Use no-added-sugar** marinara sauce, peanut butter, ketchup, and other condiments.

These changes all improve the healthfulness of meals without affecting taste or increasing meal cost. Of course, some are more challenging than others. You do not need to switch everything immediately, or even at all. Once again, this book is a collection of suggestions, not an action plan. Do what is best for your FAA.

A challenge to you: take one step towards making a meal you prepare look more like the MyPlate graphic. Baby steps equal little improvements in nutrition, and little improvements in nutrition add up to big improvements in health, wellness, and quality of life.

Chapter 11: Cost-Effectiveness

Cost is a major factor that influences food choice for anyone, but especially food assistance agencies (FAAs). Because money and food are so closely intertwined, FAAs must pay careful attention to food cost. When serving large groups of people, costs can add up where you least expect them, using up valuable funding available to purchase food. The more economical you are when planning and preparing meals, the more room in your budget you will have and the more people you can help.

Most FAAs want to save money but are also concerned with the quality of the food or meals they provide. There is a difference between *inexpensive* food and *cheap* food. Money can be saved without sacrificing the meal's flavor and acceptability. This chapter provides suggestions and tips on how to reduce plate cost. These tips are primarily targeted towards food kitchens and other FAAs that serve prepared meals, but anyone can gain something from thinking about cost-effectiveness. More clinical instructions on how to calculate plate cost can be found in resources if you are interested in the math.

Reducing Plate Cost:

Plate cost is essentially a measure of cost per serving, or how much it costs in total to serve a specific recipe to one person. Plate cost is helpful because it shows which meals are the most expensive to serve, and which ingredients are contributing the most to cost. With this information, your FAA can budget for meals and make changes to recipes in order to reduce cost.

Imagine that your FAA chooses to serve spaghetti with beef meatballs and marinara sauce. Here is the plate cost chart for this meal. The first column shows the cost of each ingredient needed to make six servings of the meal. Beside cost per ingredient is a column with the plate cost (one serving) of each ingredient.

Plate Cost of Spaghetti:

Ingredient:	Cost per recipe:	Plate cost:
Angel Hair Pasta (1 12 oz box)	$2.00	$0.33
Marinara Sauce (3 cup)	$4.99	$0.83
Meatballs (36)	$6.99	$1.17
Takeaway Box (6)	$3.15	$0.53
TOTAL:	$17.13	$2.86

For one serving with 2 oz of pasta, 1/2 cup of marinara sauce, and 6 meatballs packaged in a takeaway box (a fold over take-out food container), you will pay $2.86. That's a lot, and the cost will add up quickly. Here is what that would look like in quantity:

Spaghetti in Quantity:

10 servings	$28.60
25 servings	$71.50
50 servings	$143.00
100 servings	$286.00

Your FAA may not typically serve that many clients, but you get the picture- this recipe could take a huge bite out of your budget. Several things can reduce the price of this meal and make it more affordable.

To begin, look at the brands of ingredients used. Obviously, the initial plan included purchasing a rather pricey name-brand marinara sauce and name-brand pasta. Try transitioning to the local store-brand. Here is how ingredient cost would change:

Plate Cost of Spaghetti:

Ingredient:	Cost per recipe:	Plate cost:
Angel Hair Pasta (1 12oz box)	$1.20	$0.20
Marinara Sauce (3 cup)	$2.50	$0.50
Meatballs (36)		
Takeaway Box (6)		
TOTAL:		

Another contributor to the price is the meatballs. Meat, in general, can drastically increase plate cost, as it is usually the most expensive ingredient in a meal. Using fewer meatballs and adding some bulk by using frozen broccoli can help keep costs under control.

Plate Cost of Spaghetti:

Ingredient:	Cost per recipe:	Plate cost:
Angel Hair Pasta (1 12oz box)	$1.20	$0.20
Marinara Sauce (3 cup)	$2.50	$0.50
Meatballs (24)	$4.66	$0.78
Broccoli (3 cup)	$1.10	$0.18
Takeaway Box (6)		
TOTAL:		

$0.21 can be saved by replacing 2 meatballs with 1/2 cup of broccoli. With 4 meatballs, the meal still has a satisfying amount of meat. As a bonus, using broccoli adds some extra fiber and micronutrients to an already delicious meal.

Finally, plate cost can be reduced by eliminating packaging and using reusable plates instead of takeaway boxes. When making this decision, you will need to weigh your options. You might opt to save $0.53 by using reusable plates, or perhaps your unique situation makes disposables a necessity. For example, Small FAAs may not have access to adequate dishwashing equipment, and in that case, disposables are more sanitary. If your FAA serves exclusively to-go meals, reusables are impractical. Choose what works best for you. The example will switch to plates:

Plate Cost of Spaghetti:

Ingredient:	Cost per recipe:	Plate cost:
Angel Hair Pasta (1 12oz box)	$1.20	$0.20
Marinara Sauce (3 cup)	$2.50	$0.50
Meatballs (24)	$4.66	$0.78
Broccoli (3 cup)	$1.10	$0.18
TOTAL:	$9.46	$1.66

The final plate cost is $1.66. By switching to cheaper brands, reducing the meat, and eliminating packaging, the spaghetti and meatballs recipe's plate cost decreases from $2.86 to only $1.66 per serving. That is a difference of $1.20! How does that affect the quantity prices?

Spaghetti in Quantity:

10 servings	$16.60
25 servings	$41.50
50 servings	$83.00
100 servings	$166.00

For 100 servings, the price decreases from $286.00 to $166.00, a difference of $120.00. Using these savings, we can serve spaghetti and meatballs to *an additional 72 clients!*

As you can see, large amounts of money can be saved if you pay close attention to where cost is coming from and know how to reduce it.

Of course, reducing plate cost is only helpful if you do not sacrifice the quality of your meals, or your sanity. For example, you might taste-test the store-brand spaghetti sauce and find that it does not meet standards. Maybe you opt to spend a bit extra on name-brand or purchase additional spices to improve the flavor of the store-brand spaghetti sauce. Similarly, perhaps you have limited time to wash reusable plates after every meal and feel that takeaway boxes are worth the money to avoid hassle. Restaurants must make these decisions for their products, and so will you. Like everything else in this book, this is totally customizable to you.

Suggestions to Reduce Plate Cost:

1) **Use more meatless recipes.** Meat is often the most expensive element of a recipe. High-protein, budget-friendly alternatives to meat include eggs, beans/peas/legumes, and dairy products like yogurt.

2) **Make casseroles.** Casseroles are versatile, and there are endless flavor possibilities. Examples are breakfast casseroles with eggs, cheese, and ham/sausage, or rice casseroles with creamy sauces, vegetables, and canned chicken. Many casserole recipes use little or no meat and can be stretched by adding extra grains and veggies.

3) **Smaller portion sizes.** If you notice that clients do not finish the meal you serve, consider giving out less. Extra food can be distributed as seconds if some clients are still hungry. This helps ensure that most of the food you distribute is actually eaten.

4) **Alternative items.** Similarly, if you notice that people are not eating an item at all, switch to something new.

5) **Do not be afraid of canned and frozen foods.** Whether fresh, frozen, dried, or canned, eating more healthy food has

benefits. Preserved foods are often more affordable than their fresh counterparts.

6) **Cook in-season.** In-season foods are usually cheapest, and they taste better.

7) **Do not "scrape away your profit."** Overall, what you don't use is still worth money, so it's important to use every last bit of food as much as possible. Avoid waste.

Chapter 12: The Resources

As promised, here is a list of resources that will be helpful for several areas in a food assistance agency. For the sake of quick access and easy updates, all of these resources are available online at this webpage:

https://gatewaygaston.org/-gateway-to-nutrition/

You will find links to all the resources mentioned in each chapter, along with recipes, nutrition information, and client educational materials. Also included are some further reading that will be helpful if you want to learn more about the charitable food system, food insecurity, food deserts, food safety, and nutrition.

Chapter 13: Conclusion and Acknowledgements

Food insecurity and food deserts exist in every community, and often feel like problems that are too big to tackle. Running an FAA takes motivation, commitment, consistency, and strength, yet sometimes, it is easy to feel discouraged. But I have hope for a better tomorrow, one where everyone has access to proper nutrition. You should have this same hope because you are helping to create that better tomorrow.

Amazing people like you tirelessly strive towards a future where everyone has access to enough nutrition for a healthy, active life. I want this book to uplift, encourage, and equip you with tools and knowledge that will help your FAA thrive. From the bottom of my heart, thank you for what you do every day in your community. First and foremost, this book is for you.

My name is Laurel Davis. I am a Nutrition and Dietetics major at Carson-Newman University, a Bonner Scholar, and the Nutrition Nonprofit Support Intern at the Gateway Gaston.

The purpose of the Gateway is to connect the community of Gaston County, North Carolina, for the common good. The Gateway Gaston connects people with resources throughout our community, extending a hand-up (not just a handout) to help them create positive life change. We partner with over 100 nonprofit agencies and houses of worship, and we helped over 3,500 families get connected to resources they needed during the last calendar year.

R. Dwayne Burks is the Director and Chaplain of the Gateway Gaston. He said, on behalf of the Gateway: "This project is a labor of love from the Gateway to the community to meet a practical need. Most importantly it illustrates the importance of collaboration."

The charitable food system is made up of many diverse and unique agencies, each with its own strengths, challenges, and resources. Collaboration is essential to create meaningful progress and change. This book is a perfect example of what can happen when unique, talented, and ultimately *different* people work together. I want to introduce you to everyone who made this book possible.

While writing this book, I had the honor and privilege to meet, have conversations with, and serve alongside 13 Gateway Gaston partners. I observed the fantastic work they do every day, saw how they distribute food to the community, and learned from passionate volunteers and directors. This book was written with the needs, strengths, and challenges of these partners in mind. I want to express my gratitude to them. Without their time, hospitality, expertise, and kindness, this book would not be possible.

Thank you to my colleagues at the Gateway for everything you have done and continue to do with this book. This was truly a group project. We did this together. I have deeply enjoyed working with every one of you, and my greatest hope is that the opportunity for us to collaborate arises again in the future.

Thank you to Cox Walsh & Associates and Leslie Davis for your time and expertise editing this writing. Thank you to everyone who read earlier drafts and provided valuable feedback.

Thank you to the Greater Gaston Baptist Association. You are amazing people, doing amazing work in our community and for the Kingdom of God. I had a wonderful summer working with you and learning from you.

Thank you to Carson-Newman University, and every faculty and staff member who has poured into my education and life. Special thanks to Dr.

Beverley Hammond, who entertained my countless questions as I wrote this book.

Thank you to everyone involved in the Bonner Scholars Program at Carson-Newman University, who have helped me grow my knowledge about social justice, community, and nonprofit work. Special thanks to Dr. Matthew Bryant-Cheney, Ms. Gabby Valentine, and Mr. Alexander Nichols. Thank you to my fellow Bonner Scholars for being my second family.

Thank you to my family and future husband, Gavan White, for loving me, reminding me to enjoy life, supporting me through everything, and pretending to understand my random, avid explanations of food insecurity statistics. I love you.

I would also like to thank Dr. Katie S. Martin, Executive Director of the Foodshare Institute for Hunger Research & Solutions and the author of one of my favorite books, _Reinventing Food Banks and Pantries: New Tools to End Hunger._ Her work has influenced my passion for the charitable food system, my vision for this book, and my vision for my future career.

Thank you to Mr. Nick Grice from Real Life Church in Stanley, NC for connecting me with The

Gateway Gaston and this internship. This wonderful opportunity all began with you.

Finally, I want to thank R. Dwayne Burks, the director and chaplain of the Gateway Gaston, from the bottom of my heart. You will never know the extent to which you shaped the direction of my life. I am beyond grateful for the opportunity to intern at such an impactful organization, under such an impactful person. I hope that I can someday be a fraction of the changemaker, Christian, and person that you are.

Works Cited

"4 Steps to Food Safety.", U.S. Department of Health and Human Services, 14 Dec. 2020, www.foodsafety.gov/keep-food-safe/4-steps-to-food-safety. Accessed 26 July 2021.

"About the Atlas." U.S. Department of Agriculture, Economic Research Service, 27 Apr. 2021, www.ers.usda.gov/data-products/food-access-research-atlas/about-the-atlas.

"Are You Storing Food Safely?" US Food and Drug Administration, 9 Feb. 2021, www.fda.gov/consumers/consumer-updates/are-you-storing-food-safely. Accessed 26 July 2021.

Arnold, John. *Charity Food Programs That Can End Hunger in America.* Second Harvest Gleaners Food Bank of West Michigan, 2004, https://www.endhungerinamerica.org/publications/charity-food-programs-that-can-end-hunger-in-america/. *End Hunger in America*, Accessed 28, July 2021.

Berkowitz, Seth A., et al. "State-Level and County-Level Estimates of Health Care Costs Associated with Food Insecurity." *Preventing Chronic Disease*, vol. 16, 11 July 2019, www.cdc.gov/pcd/issues/2019/18_0549.htm, 10.5888/pcd16.180549.

"Burden of Foodborne Illness: Findings.", Centers for Disease Control and Prevention, 5 Nov. 2018, www.cdc.gov/foodborneburden/2011-foodborne-estimates.html. Accessed 28 July 2021.

Burks, Dwayne. Personal interview. 17 July 2021.

Bush-Kaufman, Alexandra, et al. "In-Depth Qualitative Interviews to Explore Healthy Environment Strategies in Food Pantries in the Western United States." *Journal of the Academy of Nutrition and Dietetics*, vol. 119, no. 10, Oct. 2019, pp. 1632–1643, 10.1016/j.jand.2019.05.010.

Chaifetz, Ashley, and Benjamin Chapman. "Evaluating North Carolina Food Pantry Food Safety-Related Operating Procedures." *Journal of Food Protection*, vol. 78, no. 11, 2015, pp. 2033-2042. *ProQuest*, doi.org/10.4315/0362-028x.jfp-15-084

"Charitable Food System." UConn Rudd Center for Food Policy & Obesity, *uconnruddcenter.org/research/foodsecurity/charitable-food/*. Accessed 27 Jul. 2021.

"Definitions of Food Security." U.S. Department of Agriculture, Economic Research Service, 9 Sept.

2020, www.ers.usda.gov/topics/food-nutrition-assistance/food-security-in-the-us/definitions-of-food-security/.

Dietary Guidelines for Americans, 2020-2025. 9th Edition. December 2020. Available at DietaryGuidelines.gov.

Dutko, Paula, Michele Ver Ploeg, and Tracey Farrigan. Characteristics and Influential Factors of Food Deserts, ERR-140, U.S. Department of Agriculture, Economic Research Service, August 2012.

"Food Access Research Atlas." U.S. Department of Agriculture, Economic Research Service, 27 Apr. 2021 https://www.ers.usda.gov/data-products/food-access-research-atlas/

"Food Product Dating." *U.S. Department of Agriculture Food Safety and Inspection Service*, 2 Oct. 2019, www.fsis.usda.gov/food-safety/safe-food-handling-and-preparation/food-safety-basics/food-product-dating. Accessed 26 July 2021.

"Food Security in the U.S." U.S. Department of Agriculture, Economic Research Service, 12 Mar. 2021, www.ers.usda.gov/topics/food-nutrition-assistance/food-security-in-the-us/.

Gundersen, C., Strayer, M., Dewey, A., Hake, M., & Engelhard, E. (2021). *Map the Meal Gap 2021: An Analysis of County and Congressional District Food Insecurity and County Food Cost in the United States in 2019.* Feeding America.

Hammond, Beverley. Personal interview. 3 Aug. 2021.

"Handwashing: A Healthy Habit in the Kitchen." *Www.cdc.gov,* U.S. Centers for Disease Control and Prevention, 6 May 2021, www.cdc.gov/handwashing/handwashing-kitchen.html. Accessed 26 July 2021.

"Healthcare Costs of Food Insecurity, The." Feeding America Research. *Tableau Public,* 19 June 2019, public.tableau.com/app/profile/feeding.america.research/viz/TheHealthcareCostsofFoodInsecurity/HealthcareCosts. Accessed 26 July 2021.

Martin, Katie S. *Reinventing Food Banks and Pantries: New Tools to End Hunger.* Washington, DC, Island Press, 9 Mar. 2021.

Martin, Katie S., et al. "Supporting Wellness at Pantries: Development of a Nutrition Stoplight System for Food Banks and Food Pantries." *Journal of the Academy of Nutrition and Dietetics,* vol. 119, no. 4, Apr. 2019, p. 553. *EBSCOhost,* doi:10.1016/j.jand.2018.03.003

"MyPlate." *MyPlate.gov*, 2021, www.myplate.gov/. Accessed 26 July 2021.

"Nutrition." *Merriam-Webster.com Dictionary*, Merriam-Webster, https://www.merriam-webster.com/dictionary/nutrition. Accessed 16 Aug. 2021.

Ohio Association of Second Harvest Foodbanks. *Making the Switch: A Guide for Converting to a Client Choice Food Pantry.* https://secure3.convio.net/fdshr/site/DocServer/Switching_to_Choice_Pantry_-_Ohio.pdf

Pritt, Laura A., et al. "Barriers Confronting Food Pantry Clients: Lack of Kitchen Supplies: A Pilot Study." *Social Work and Christianity*, vol. 45, no. 2, 2018, pp. 68-85. *ProQuest*, proquest.com/scholarly-journals/barriers-confronting-food-pantry-clients-lack/docview/2135990013/se-2?accountid=9900.

"Recalls and Outbreaks.", U.S. Department of Health & Human Services, 13 Jan. 2020, www.foodsafety.gov/recalls-and-outbreaks. Accessed 26 July 2021.

"Refrigeration & Food Safety.", U.S. Department of Agriculture, 23 Mar. 2015, www.fsis.usda.gov/food-safety/safe-food-handling-and-preparation/food-safety-basics/refrigeration. Accessed 26 July 2021.

"Safe Minimum Internal Temperature Chart." U.S Department of Agriculture, 11 May 2020, www.fsis.usda.gov/food-safety/safe-food-handling-and-preparation/food-safety-basics/safe-temperature-chart. Accessed 26 July 2021.

Seligman, Hilary K., and Dean Schillinger. "Hunger and Socioeconomic Disparities in Chronic Disease." *New England Journal of Medicine*, vol. 363, no. 1, 1 July 2010, pp. 6–9, www.nejm.org/doi/full/10.1056/NEJMp1000072, 10.1056/nejmp1000072. Accessed 26 July 2021.

"Shelf-Stable Food Safety." U.S. Department of Agriculture, 24 Mar. 2015, www.fsis.usda.gov/food-safety/safe-food-handling-and-preparation/food-safety-basics/shelf-stable-food. Accessed 26 July 2021.

"Surplus, Salvaged, and Donated Foods." US Food and Drug Administration, 30 Oct. 2017, www.fda.gov/food/buy-store-serve-safe-food/surplus-salvaged-and-donated-foods. Accessed 26 July 2021.

Thomas, Jeff. *How to Run a Food Pantry*. Second Harvest Gleaners Food Bank of West Michigan, 2007,

https://www.endhungerinamerica.org/publications/
how-to-run-a-food-pantry/. *End Hunger in America*,
Accessed 28, July 2021.

Waite, Tori. "What's the Difference between a Food Bank
and Food Pantry?" Feeding America, 20 Feb. 2019,
www.feedingamerica.org/hunger-blog/what-
difference-between-food-bank-and-food-pantry.
Accessed 27 Jul. 2021

Weinfield, Nancy S, et al. "Hunger in America 2014
National Report." Feeding America, 2014.

"What Is Cross-Contamination?" U.S. Department of
Agriculture, AskUSDA, 17 July 2019,
ask.usda.gov/s/article/What-is-Cross-
Contamination. Accessed 3 Aug. 2021.